ASK DR. WEIL

HEALTHY
LIVING

By Andrew Weil, M.D.:

HEALTHY LIVING

Andrew Weil, M.D.

Edited by Steven Petrow

IVY BOOKS • NEW YORK

All material provided in the Ask Dr. Weil program is provided for educational purposes only. Consult your own physician regarding the applicability of any opinions or recommendations with respect to your symptoms or medical condition.

Questions contained in this book may appear in other volumes of the Ask Dr. Weil series. The books are arranged according to topic, and to create a complete health profile utilizing Dr. Weil's prescriptions, material may overlap.

Ivy Books
Published by Ballantine Books
Copyright © 1997 by Great Bear Productions, LLC.

ISBN 0-8041-1673-3

Manufactured in the United States of America

Introduction

You've taken the first step toward optimum health. This book will give you more information about my philosophy along with answers to some of the questions I am asked most frequently.

I wrote *Spontaneous Healing* and *8 Weeks to Optimum Health* because I wanted to call attention to the innate, intrinsic nature of the healing process. I've always believed that the body can heal itself if you give it a chance. Why? Because it has a healing system. If you're feeling well, you will want to know about this system so that you can enhance your well-being. If you are ill, you'll also want to know about it because it is your best hope of recovery.

To maintain optimum health requires commitment. This book—and the others in the series—can give you much of the basic information you need about diet, supplements, common illnesses, natural remedies, and healthy living.

All of these questions originated on "Ask Dr. Weil," my program on the World Wide Web. If you still have questions, come visit the clinic at www.drweil.com.

Do I Need
Abs of Steel?

Q:

It seems that I can't turn on the television anymore without seeing an infomercial for an abdominal exercising gizmo. Are any of these products really effective at helping a person "lose inches" and "shape the midsection"?

A:

Let me say at the start that washboard stomachs aren't necessarily desirable. Sure, they look good on slick magazine paper (and the TV screen), but they may not be healthy. A super-flat abdomen with tight, rippling muscles will restrict the motion of the intestines during digestion. It may also crimp the action of the diaphragm, which needs to move freely in order for you to breathe optimally. It's okay to be trim, but a well-toned abdomen should be yielding, not rigid.

The ab-gizmo makers are just the latest industry to capitalize on our society's obsession with lean bodies. In 1995, they sold $145 million worth of these devices.

Abdominal crunches in moderation can be helpful. They can strengthen the back as well as the abdominal muscles. They help reduce back pain by balancing and toning the muscles that support the spine. And they may help some people shape their midsections.

You don't need to buy an expensive apparatus to work your abdominal muscles: a basic stomach crunch will do. Lie on the floor with knees bent, palms on your legs or on the floor, and feet comfortably apart. Keep your chin up (focus your eyes on the ceiling) and curl your body forward until your shoulders are a few inches off the floor. Hold, relax, and repeat. And remember to keep breathing.

It does make sense to pay attention to your body weight. If you are more than 20 percent heavier than your ideal weight, you may have increased risk of cardiovascular disease, diabetes, gallstones, some kinds of cancer, and osteoarthritis. Also note that body composition may be a more accurate way to determine your ideal weight than actuarial tables. Percentage of body fat is usually measured by weighing under water, but new computerized analysis is much simpler—and drier!

Remember: Spot reduction isn't the answer, whether you use those devices or not. The secret to losing weight won't cost you anything: eat less (especially less fat) and get more aerobic exercise. If you want to crunch your abs, that's okay, too.

Is Aspartame Dangerous?

Q:

I think I've had an adverse reaction to aspartame. I've used NutraSweet for fifteen years, usually consuming six to eight packets a day. Now I have reduced motor control of my arms and hands. Is there a link? What do you recommend?

A:

First of all, I would stop using NutraSweet. Although the manufacturer portrays aspartame as a gift from nature, and its two components do occur naturally, aspartame itself does not. Like all artificial sweeteners, aspartame has a peculiar taste. Because I have seen a number of patients—mostly women— who report headaches from using it, I don't view it as biologically inert. Some women also find that aspartame aggravates PMS. There are no proven long-term toxic effects, but there is a lot of suspicion.

In general, I think you're better off using moderate amounts of sugar. People who use NutraSweet to control their weight should know there's not a shred of evidence that the availability or use of artificial sweeteners has helped anyone to lose weight. Think about it: You have pie à la mode for dessert (about 495 calories), and then use a packet of NutraSweet for your coffee (saving 18 calories). There's something wrong with that calculation. Also, remember that aspartame turns up in unexpected items. Recently, on an airplane, I was given some mints that were sweetened with aspartame. Most people wouldn't have noticed it in the fine print on the label.

As for your motor troubles, I would advise going to a

neurologist for an evaluation. Your condition may be unrelated to aspartame, although there is some anecdotal evidence indicating a link.

How Safe Are Barbecues?

Q:
Our family is planning a couple of BBQs. Are there dangers to grilling?

A:
We know that charcoal grilling produces carcinogenic smoke from the high-temperature cooking of foods containing fat and protein (hot dogs, hamburgers, and chicken to name some of your likely favorites) and unhealthy chemical changes in the outer layers of flesh foods. My two top recommendations: Don't inhale, and get used to cutting off any black or charred parts. Also, new research indicates that marinating meats for four hours greatly reduces their carcinogenicity on the grill.

Never use charcoal-lighting fluid or those self-lighting packages of charcoal; they both put residues from toxic chemicals into the food. I always use a "chimney lighter," in which a small amount of newspaper is ignited to get the coals burning.

I've noticed the trend toward more gourmet barbecuing—specifically, with mesquite briquettes. They're no better or worse than conventional briquettes, and the market for them is decimating the mesquite forests of the Southwest. On the other hand, I read recently that more people than ever before are using gas grills. That's good news for the environment.

By the way, fish or vegetables are great when grilled. Here's a recipe I often use.

Grilled Vegetables

Make a marinade of equal parts sake (or dry vermouth),
olive oil, and Japanese soy sauce (shoyu). Add a few
mashed garlic cloves and some hot pepper sauce if desired.
Cut vegetables (onions, carrots, mushrooms, zucchini, red
and green peppers, eggplants) into bite-size pieces and toss
in the marinade to coat well. Let sit for thirty minutes while
the grill is heating. Drain veggies and thread on skewers in
artful order, then grill till they become tender and begin to
brown. Serve with rice.

Crippled by Carpal Tunnel Syndrome?

Q:
Due to repetitive typing I have developed carpal tunnel syndrome in both arms. I was given anti-inflammatory medication for this. Then I developed stomach problems—gastritis and irritable bowel syndrome. I recently have begun to see a doctor of Eastern medicine, who started me on herbs including ginger tablets with DGL (deglycyrrhizinated licorice). On my second visit he performed acupuncture. Do you think that with Eastern medicine my carpal tunnel will also get better?

A:
When you're an especially speedy typist or spend long hours at the keyboard, the tendons that move the fingers can swell. There's one little tunnel through the ligament at the base of your palm that all the tendons and one very important nerve pass through from your arm to your hand. That's where the swelling can cause pressure and pain, the condition known as carpal tunnel syndrome (CTS).

The most effective treatment that I've found is vitamin B-6 (pyridoxine), 100 milligrams, two or three times a day. In this dosage, pyridoxine is not acting as a B vitamin but rather as a natural therapeutic agent that relieves nerve compression injuries. Be aware that doses of B-6 higher than 300 milligrams a day have caused rare cases of nerve damage. Discontinue usage if you develop any unusual numbness. (A much-publicized University of Michigan study warned about nerve toxicity with B-6 and discouraged people from using it for CTS. I disagree.)

For quick relief when you're hurting, rub on arnica gel, which you can find in your health food store or drugstore. Also, try wrapping ice packs around your wrists (a bag of frozen peas works just as well); if you use this treatment for five minutes every few hours when you're especially stressing your wrists, it may ease the pain and the inflammation. The ginger you mention may relieve inflammation over time, and acupuncture certainly can provide symptomatic relief.

The most important consideration when you've got CTS is to figure out ways to reduce the repetitive strain. Unless you do so, long-term improvement is unlikely. That means doing less typing, and learning how to stop driving yourself so hard at the keyboard. Here are a few other tips: Make yourself stand up every hour for a few minutes and stretch. The muscles in your wrists are connected to those in your arms, shoulders, and neck. Pay attention to those parts of your body, too, because stretching and relaxing your shoulders, neck, and back can ease the strain on your wrists. I know some people who have found relief through deep-tissue massage or Rolfing. And consider whether you're feeling emotional tension at work that can tighten your whole body, making it more susceptible to injury.

Your posture at the keyboard can make a big difference. Sit up straight, with your weight slightly forward. Your feet should be flat on the floor, or tilted comfortably on an adjustable footrest. An adjustable keyboard tray will allow you to change the position of your hands now and then, and keep your wrists straight, with your forearms horizontal and at a 90-degree angle to your upper arms. Your elbows should be at your sides in a relaxed position. Every now and then, tilt your head slowly to each side, and roll your shoulders twice forward and twice back. Squeeze your hands into tight fists, and then stretch your fingers out as wide as they will go. Close your hands into fists again and rotate your wrists a few times in either direction.

You might also try a different keyboard. Each brand has its own key touches and key widths, some of which may feel better to you than others. If you can find a split keyboard, it may help you keep your hands and arms at a more natural angle. There are also some new keyboards with concave keys, sections tilted up like an accordion, and other unusual shapes. I haven't tried them, but you may want to check them out.

Killing Me Softly
with Your Cloves?

Q:
How bad for you are clove cigarettes compared to regular cigarettes? I've read conflicting reports and have heard that one clove cigarette is equivalent to smoking an entire pack of regular cigarettes. Please give me your advice.

A:
Sometimes people mistakenly assume that clove cigarettes are healthier than regular cigarettes because cloves are more "natural," but those people must not have read the labels. Clove cigarettes are just tobacco with clove flavor. That may mean tobacco mixed with cloves, but often it means tobacco mixed with artificial clove flavoring and other fragrances. Clove cigarettes are also usually unfiltered, and they may deliver three times as much tar as a regular Marlboro.

Still, I can't believe that smoking one clove cigarette is equivalent to smoking an entire pack of regular cigarettes. But clove cigarette smoke can be more irritating than the smoke of regular cigarettes, depending on individual sensitivity.

Everything we know regarding secondhand smoke and tobacco is applicable to clove cigarettes because of the tobacco in them. Plus, to me, the smoke smells worse than plain tobacco smoke. I'm not sure of all the health risks of inhaling components of clove oil on a regular basis, but there are reported cases of allergic pneumonitis (inflammation of the lungs) in people who smoke clove cigarettes.

Expired Contact Lenses?

Q:
Why do my disposable contact lenses have an expiration date? Is it dangerous to wear them beyond that date?

A:
It's really important to follow manufacturers' instructions about contact lenses. That thin piece of plastic that helps you see sits directly on your eye. About half the 18.2 million contact lens wearers in the United States use soft lenses, which are especially likely to cause infection if special handling techniques aren't followed. The plastic can become brittle over time, and the lenses can become carriers for bacteria. You should return or throw away lenses that have expired.

Two organisms, *Pseudomonas aeruginosa* and *Acanthamoeba castellanii*, are especially associated with infections of the cornea from poor contact lens hygiene. People like you who wear disposable lenses are at highest risk for infection. In one study, people who used disposable daily-wear lenses had a 49 percent higher risk of *Acanthamoeba* infection than those who wore conventional soft lenses. The most common reasons for infection were failure to disinfect the lenses and use of chlorine-release lens disinfection systems, which aren't effective against that particular organism.

Even if you wear lenses approved for overnight wear, don't keep them on overnight. With that kind of usage, there is a much greater chance of damaging the cornea and allowing bacteria to build up.

Is Decaf Really
Any Better?

Q:
How much safer is decaf than regular coffee?

A:
Although new caffeine extraction methods seem to preserve the flavor of a good cup of coffee, decaffeinated coffee is not necessarily the answer for java junkies. Decaf retains enough caffeine to affect sensitive individuals. It also contains other substances naturally found in the coffee bean that can have irritating effects on the body. For example, decaffeinated coffee can be just as rough on the stomach as regular coffee.

If you have reason to avoid coffee, you would do well to avoid decaf also. If you have any of the following conditions, stay away from both drinks: migraine, tremor, anxiety, irregular heartbeat, insomnia, coronary heart disease or a strong family history of it, high cholesterol, any gastrointestinal disorder, any urinary disorder, prostate trouble, fibrocystic breasts, premenstrual syndrome, tension headaches, or seizure disorder.

A study done at the University of California at Berkeley found a relationship between drinking decaf and a slightly increased risk of high cholesterol and heart disease. In that survey of about 45,500 men, regular coffee did not have the same effect.

If you really want to drink decaf, I'd recommend using only the water-extracted versions. There is concern that traces of solvents may remain in coffee decaffeinated by other methods, although the manufacturers deny it.

There are many coffee substitutes available in supermarkets and health food stores. They are made from roasted grains, roots, acorns, and other benign ingredients. I recommend Cafix, Roma, Dacopa, and Teccino. Experiment with them, or use a caffeine-free herbal tea.

E. coli in the Apple Juice?

Q:

I'm worried about drinking E. coli*–infected apple juice. How does this happen? What can I do to protect myself from* E. coli*? What are the symptoms—and remedies?*

A:

You are right to be worried. A 1996 outbreak of *E. coli* poisoning from Odwalla Company apple juice focused attention on the dangers of unpasteurized juice—a product we thought was as wholesome as apple pie. This outbreak came just weeks after a similar one in Connecticut, where 10 people were made ill by unpasteurized apple cider. In both cases, it appears that the juice manufacturers followed all recommended guidelines that apples be brushed and washed before being pressed into juice.

"E. coli" is an abbreviation for *Escherichia coli* bacteria— a mostly harmless germ that lives in the intestines of humans and animals; it helps its hosts by suppressing the growth of harmful bacteria and by synthesizing important vitamins. But in recent years, a virulent strain known as *E. coli* 0157:H7 has made headlines in a number of food-poisoning outbreaks around the world. This latest outbreak, traced to California apples, was small compared to other episodes.

In 1993, undercooked, fecally contaminated hamburgers from Jack-in-the Box killed 4 people and sickened some 700 others. In 1996 in Japan, more than 9,000 people were sickened by a similar strain. *E. coli*–infected apple juice was never considered a real possibility until a 1991 outbreak was traced to cider pressed in Massachusetts. According to the FDA, *E. coli* 0157:H7 is evolving and "has adapted to survive in a more acidic environment," such as unpasteurized apple cider.

E. coli infection occurs primarily in two ways. Bacteria can leak from animals' intestines into meat intended for human consumption. Or *E. coli* can be present in completely un-cooked foods, such as juice. Illness from *E. coli* has also been traced to consumption of salami, deli roast beef, raw milk, lake water, mayonnaise, cantaloupe, and leafy vegetables like lettuce.

Infection often causes stomach cramps and bloody diarrhea several hours to several days after ingestion. There may be slight fever and possibly vomiting. Generally, the illness resolves in five to ten days, but in children under five and the elderly, the infection can cause hemolytic uremia syndrome (HUS), in which red blood cells are destroyed and the kidneys fail. This complication occurs in 2 to 7 percent of cases and can be fatal.

With juice, it's always difficult to pinpoint the source of contamination. Often apple juice is made from "groundfall" or "drop" apples. When that juice is unpasteurized, any con-taminants from the manure of grazing cows or deer—or from farm runoff—that are not completely washed off can get into the juice during pressing. Federal authorities are consider-ing new requirements that juice shipped interstate be pasteur-ized. An alternative would be to test juice for the presence of *E. coli*.

If you're concerned, you can bring unpasteurized juice to a rolling boil, which will kill any lingering microorganisms. To protect yourself from *E. coli* infection from meat, wash your hands and all cutting surfaces thoroughly after handling raw meat, and be sure to cook meat to 160°.

As for treatment, there is little evidence that antibiotics help (they may increase risk of kidney complications). Anti-diarrheal agents should also be avoided. Time is usually the best treatment. HUS, however, is life-threatening, requiring intensive care in a hospital. If you have any reason to suspect you've ingested contaminated juice (or other foods) and are having symptoms, call your doctor or local health department.

Could I Really Use an Enema?

Q:

I read your book Spontaneous Healing *and found it absolutely marvelous. I was, however, surprised that you never mentioned enemas or colonics as an adjunctive therapy for detoxification. I know the Gerson therapy and other alternative cancer treatments make extensive use of these measures. What is your opinion about them?*

A:

Enemas enjoyed great popularity in the seventeenth and eighteenth centuries, when they were considered both fashionable and medically necessary. Louis XIV of France was quite an enthusiast, sometimes undergoing as many as four a day—often during meetings with dignitaries. At that time, people believed that constipation resulted from "hypochondriacal melancholy," a problem that afflicted only the most noble and intelligent men. Similar symptoms in women were associated with "hysteria," in which the overheated womb wandered through the body longing for fulfillment. Mayan shamans took hallucinogenic enemas; made with mead, tobacco juice, mushrooms, and morning glory seeds, the enemas must have induced massively altered states of consciousness.

Proponents of enemas today argue that they clean away microorganisms, impacted feces, and dead cells while relieving constipation, backache, fatigue, headache, loss of concentration, and other maladies. Quite a list. Colonic irrigation involves flushing the entire colon with running water.

The Gerson therapy you mention uses coffee enemas, plus a

special juice diet, as a treatment for cancer. Its purpose is to detoxify the body and restore normal function to poisoned cells, which then mobilize to fight tumors. Coffee by this route is stimulating and addictive, claims of enthusiasts notwithstanding. Whether coffee enemas really detoxify the liver or any other organ is an open question. I don't think there is any health need for enemas and colonics, despite their interesting history. The best way to ensure the health and normal cleanliness of the colon is to make sure you're having regular eliminations: eat a diet that's high in fiber, drink enough water, and get adequate exercise. Avoid putting things into you that are toxic in the first place. The colon sheds its entire lining and regenerates it every day, so it's impossible for anything to build up on its walls.

To increase your fiber intake, you can eat psyllium seed husks in a variety of forms. There's also an herbal bowel-regulator called Triphala, from the Ayurvedic tradition, that is very effective. You can get it from a health food store; follow the dosage recommendations on the label.

A short "fruit fast" can give your digestive system a rest. I've done a ten-day regimen that included two days of fresh fruit, two days of fruit juice, two days of water only, then two days of fruit juice, and finally two days of fruit. All along, I took a tablespoonful of powdered psyllium seed husks stirred into a big glass of water every day to give the intestines bulk.

Enemas and colonics are trendy, in part because there is an element of pleasure in them. That's fine as long as people are honest about it. You can become addicted to the sensation of colonics, and doing them addictively is not healthy. There's some risk of getting hepatitis or a perforated colon from them, but I think it's pretty small.

To Fast or Not to Fast to Lose Weight?

Q:

Is fasting an effective diet tactic? What are the best method and duration for a fast? What other sorts of health benefits or detriments are involved?

A:

Fasting is absolutely not an effective diet tool, because it will alter your metabolism in a direction that actually makes it harder to shed pounds. Most people, when they go back to eating, compensate by upping their consumption of calories.

There are benefits to fasting for purposes other than weight loss. (By fasting, I mean taking in nothing other than water or herbal teas. Restricting yourself to fruits, fruit juices, or other liquids can be helpful, but not in exactly the same way as fasting.) I have experimented with fasting one day a week and find it a useful physical and psychological discipline. I experience mental clarity and increased energy after a short-term fast.

Short-term fasting—up to three days—is a good home remedy for colds, flus, and toxic conditions. Combine it with rest and good mental states. Drink plenty of water to help flush out your system, and remember to stay warm and conserve your energy. Break your fast with light, plain foods.

Long-term fasting—more than three days—can also be beneficial, but it is potentially dangerous, so do not attempt it without expert supervision. It is a drastic technique. I know people who have fasted from one to three months and achieved complete remission of diseases that resisted all other treatments (bronchial asthma, rheumatoid arthritis, ulcerative colitis). Unfortunately, the diseases often return when eating resumes.

Trawling for Help on Fish Oil

Q:
We've heard such varied opinions on fish-oil supplements that we want your opinion. Help!

A:
Fish oil is probably the most important dietary source of omega-3 fatty acids, which are vital nutrients. These fatty acids reduce inflammation, protect against the abnormal clotting associated with heart attacks, inhibit cancer, and protect brain function. There may be other benefits, too: a 1992 study published in the journal *Lancet*, for example, suggested that omega-3 fatty acids prolong pregnancy by a few days and improve birthweights.

However, I don't recommend that people take fish-oil supplements to reap the benefits of omega-3s. The oils used for commercial capsules may have toxic contaminants. Also, it's not clear that the isolated fish oils reproduce the benefits of actually eating fish.

It would be much better to eat two to three servings a week of fish that contain omega-3 fatty acids. These are the oily fish from cold Northern waters: sardines, herring, mackerel, and wild salmon, which has more omega-3s than farmed salmon.

If you are vegetarian or don't like fish, the best source of omega-3s is flaxseed. You can buy the whole seeds very cheaply in health food stores, or you can order packages of golden flax seeds (with a grinder) from Heintzman Farms (see Other Resources, page 80). Keep them in the refrigerator, and grind a half cup or so at a time in a blender or coffee grinder.

Sprinkle a tablespoonful of the resulting meal onto salads, baked potatoes, or cereals. As a daily supplement, this will give you plenty of omega-3s. And it tastes good: sweet and nutty.

Be aware that flax has a very high fiber content, so it can increase stool bulk and have a laxative effect. Most people find this welcome.

To Fluoridate
or Not?

Q:

My town is going to put fluoride in our drinking water. I don't feel good about this. What do you think?

A:

I'm aware of all the arguments for and against fluoride, and I can only conclude that this is primarily an emotional issue that does not lend itself to rational discussion. I've heard everything from concerns that it may cause bone cancer to the complaint that it's a government plot to destroy people's brains.

More than half the drinking water in this country is fluoridated (meaning small amounts of fluoride are added in order to strengthen teeth and reduce cavities). There are data supporting this use; a study in the late 1980s concluded that cavities decreased by 25 percent among children in communities with fluoridated water.

You don't want more than 2 parts per million of fluoride in your drinking water, however. More than that can cause chronic, low-level fluoride poisoning, especially since many people are also using dental products that contain fluoride. If your water is fluoridated, don't use more than a pea-sized bit of any fluoride toothpaste on your brush. Too much of this element may make your teeth mottled and chalky white in places, a condition known as fluorosis (this condition afflicts mostly children).

Great excesses of fluoride can cause weight loss, brittle bones, anemia, and weakness. And some data do suggest increased cancer risk. All in all, the scientific information is contradictory, fueling the controversy rather than settling it. For example, some studies indicate that fluoridation of water contributes to hip fractures in older men and women, but other studies show no such effect.

If you're concerned about fluoride in your drinking water, filter it out. You can do this by using any of the water purifying systems—reverse osmosis and distillation, for example—that remove minerals (see page 75). If you decide to do this, however, I'd recommend that you give growing children supplemental fluoride to protect their teeth. Talk to your dentist for help with that.

Obviously, overdoses of fluoride are toxic. But in low doses, I believe, the benefits for children's teeth are immeasurable.

How Hazardous Are Food Dyes?

Q:
What's up with Yellow No. 5? I've heard rumors that it contains pig blood, and I am trying to eliminate animal products from my diet.

A:
There is no need for artificial dyes in food. They're put in purely for the convenience of manufacturers. You don't use dyes when you cook at home, so why would you want them in foods you buy? I suggest going through your pantry and throwing out anything that's got artificial color in it. That will be noted on the label as "certified color," "artificial color," or something specific like "FD & C Yellow No. 5" or "Red No. something."

Here's why: Compounds that reflect specific wavelengths of light are energetic molecules that can interact with DNA, potentially causing mutations. Many dyes that were considered safe have since been found to be carcinogenic. They might also weaken our immune systems and speed up aging. Even though artificial dyes have to get approval from the U.S. Food and Drug Administration (and similar agencies in other countries), there's no agreement from country to country as to which ones are safe.

The number you see indicates that the FDA has approved the dye for use in food, drug, and cosmetic products. FD & C Yellow No. 5 is tartrazine, a synthetic dye made from precursor organic compounds with no connection to pig blood. Tartrazine may cause allergies and hyperactivity in children. The

25

FDA has estimated that 50,000 to 100,000 Americans are sensitive to tartrazine and suffer reactions like swelling, asthma, or contact dermatitis. Several hundred products contain the dye, including drugs, cake mixes, lime and lemon beverages, cheese dishes, and fruit-flavored candies. The dye is also used in fabrics.

As a vegetarian, you don't need to worry that food dyes are of animal origin. They are all synthetic chemicals. Their main danger is their carcinogenic potential.

The color of foods contributes to the pleasure of eating. But you don't need artificial colors to enjoy your food. Even though synthetic dyes are so common, I suggest trying hard to avoid them. Natural coloring agents exist and should be used more. Annatto is an orange one made from the seed of a tropical tree and widely used to make margarine yellow and cheese orange. Chlorella is a green pigment derived from algae. Caramel (from burnt sugar) and beet extract are also common. Commercial foods containing them are okay.

How Hazardous
Are Hair Dyes?

Q:

Is it safe to use hair dyes regularly?

A:

In general, I discourage people from using hair dyes. Artificial colors are suspect in cosmetic products, just as they are in food. When you apply hair dyes to your head, they are absorbed through the scalp into the many blood vessels that supply it. There is suspicion that hair dyes can increase risk of bladder cancer, because when they are absorbed, they concentrate in the bladder. Dark dyes are of particular concern, because they contain more chemicals than light ones.

I was surprised to learn that about half of all women in the United States dye their hair—an increase of about 50 percent in the past decade. And the hair-dye market for middle-aged men is expected to grow rapidly—already one in eight men between the ages of thirteen and seventy uses dyes. Commercial hair-dye makers sell $7 billion worth of their products worldwide every year.

The most recent research on hair dyes and cancer, a seven-year study of 573,369 women by the American Cancer Society, didn't find a significantly increased risk. Women who used very dark dyes over a period of twenty years or more did show a greater tendency to develop bone cancer and non-Hodgkin's lymphoma, however. It has been suggested that dyes could have been a cause of Jacqueline Onassis's cancer. And other studies *have* associated an increased risk of cancer with hair dyes.

Cancer or no, dyes aren't very healthy for your hair. They

can cause it to become brittle and to break easily. Curiously, hair dyes aren't subject to Food and Drug Administration requirements for safety testing; they were exempted in 1938.

I would stay away from chemical dyes. If you use them, make sure you don't leave them on your head any longer than necessary. Rinse your scalp thoroughly with water when you're done. Wear gloves during the whole process.

Henna, a plant-derived dye, is okay to use. And you can find other natural dyes in health food stores. I would stick with those.

Holistic Medicine
for the People?

Q:
Natural medicine has become the upper-middle-class rage. Dr. Deepak Chopra charges thousands of dollars for his seminars. We have a doctor here in Maine who is a famous holistic practitioner for women, but won't take Medicaid patients. It costs $1,000 to be taught transcendental meditation. How and when are we going to provide alternative medicine to the poor?

A:
That's a very good question. You're quite correct that alternative medicine is available mostly to the affluent, and until insurance companies see the wisdom of paying practitioners, I think it will be hard to change the situation.

Be aware, however, that doctors like myself always try to provide patients with information about managing common ailments on their own with therapies that are cost-effective and easily available. Many elements of natural medicine are not expensive. Breathing exercises, dietary adjustment, and the use of herbs are all low-cost ways to better health. Even special treatments like acupuncture may cost much less than mainstream ones.

Some insurance companies are realizing they can save money by offering to pay for alternative care. And some groups of patients and health practitioners are lobbying for better coverage. A 1993 Harvard Medical School report found that Americans were making almost as many visits to alternative caregivers as to conventional physicians. A study by the American Western Life Insurance Company that compared conventional treatment to alternative care demonstrated some striking cost savings.

American Western Life, in Foster City, California, maintains a special plan that covers alternative care by naturopaths and specialists including acupuncturists, hypnotherapists, reflexologists, and experts in herbal medicine. It has a twenty-four-hour advice hotline for herbal remedies. Alternative Health Insurance Services, a health maintenance organization in Thousand Oaks, California, also covers a range of approaches, from Ayurvedic to traditional Chinese medicine. Blue Cross of Washington & Alaska, based in Mountlake Terrace, Washington, is creating an alternative medicine benefit plan, as is Oxford Health Plans in the Northeast. In the state of Washington, health plans are required by law to provide access to licensed chiropractors, acupuncturists, and naturopaths. Shop around: you may find insurance companies that are starting to include natural medicine in their plans.

How to Get Unleaded?

Q:

My son has lead poisoning. What will the treatment be?

A:

Lead poisoning of fetuses and young children is a serious problem in the United States. Even low-level lead exposure can cause hyperactivity, learning disabilities, and growth problems over time. High levels of lead can reduce intelligence, cause severe retardation, and even lead to early death. It's very important to test for lead in young children because they are so susceptible to its effects, particularly as their brains develop. Plus, there is so much lead in the environment that it is easy for them to get exposed. If your drinking water contains more than 10 parts per billion of lead, you and your family can consume enough of this heavy metal to cause problems.

The most common sources of lead are water from lead pipes, flakes of lead paint in older homes, lead glazes on pottery, and lead from older processing equipment and fuels that ends up in canned vegetables. Get rid of all known sources of lead. You should find out what your pipes are made of and get your water tested for lead content. Or you can purchase a home purifying system (see page 75) that will remove lead and other heavy metals. The Centers for Disease Control and Prevention suggests that every child under age six be tested for lead poisoning.

I recommend two precautions to reduce the chance of ingesting lead from household water. First, let the water run from the tap for three to five minutes after any period of nonuse. Second, don't draw water from the hot tap—even for

31

cooking—because hot water leaches out impurities much more readily than cold, and because it is likely to have picked up impurities from the hot-water tank. (No matter what your pipes are made of, water from the hot tap is unfit for human consumption.)

If you detect lead poisoning early, there are effective ways to treat it. The American Association of Naturopathic Physicians recommends a nutritional approach. The antioxidants—vitamins A, C, and E, plus selenium—can help detoxify the body and protect nerve tissue from damage. Zinc and vitamin C help reduce harm from the lead, and vitamin A may counter infections that lead-poisoned children tend to suffer. The association also suggests a regimen of herbs and amino acids to detoxify the liver.

If lead poisoning is confirmed, I would be inclined to go for conventional treatment: chelation therapy. Injected or oral chelating agents bond with lead, allowing the child to excrete the metal in the urine. The newest oral medicine is Succimer, or DMSA. The treatment normally lasts nineteen days and should go no longer than three weeks. Side effects of chelation therapy can include rash, nausea, and a loss of appetite, but the benefits of getting the lead out are much greater than the risks of therapy.

Healing with Magnets?

Q:
A member of my family consulted a healer regarding her general health, and was given magnets in order to correct her magnetic field. She is to place the left foot on one magnet and the right foot on a different magnet every day. The healer told her that this will correct imbalances caused by strong electromagnetic fields such as the ones in New York's subway system. Is this use of magnets safe, and can it be beneficial?

A:
Magnet therapy is growing in popularity after a long history rooted in the ancient cultures of China, India, and Egypt. There are various theories on the effects of magnets on the body and all sorts of claims as to their power. Roger Coghill, a British scientist, theorizes that magnets affect the iron in red blood cells, improving the blood's oxygen-carrying ability. Others say magnets stimulate nerve endings and modify electrical processes in the body. They suggest that magnets can help counteract electromagnetic pollution from devices like microwave ovens and television sets (and the New York subway system, I suppose). Frankly, we don't know a lot about the positive or negative medical effects of magnets and magnetic fields. Researchers are just beginning to explore this area.

People use magnets to relieve pain, accelerate healing, and boost mental and physical energy. For example, to relieve a toothache, magnet devotees will place the north magnetic pole of a magnet against the cheek for fifteen to twenty minutes. Putting the north pole on the forehead between your eyebrows for ten minutes at bedtime is supposed to lead to better sleep after a few days.

A number of Japanese magnetic devices are available for relief of pain, such as the pain of arthritis. You can buy magnet insoles, magnet mattress pads, magnet car-seat covers, and small magnets to place on various parts of your body. I've met patients who swear by them, but I don't think we can assume that wearing magnets is necessarily healthful—or helpful. Also, these devices are quite expensive.

Some people say that while contact with a south magnetic pole is relaxing, contact with a north magnetic pole can be stimulating and might activate latent tumors or other disease processes. Until the new field of energy medicine really gets going, I think we'll have to experiment on our own and watch for results of studies as they appear. For an overview of the subject written by an enthusiast, look up *Discovery of Magnetic Health: A Health Care Alternative* by George J. Washnis and Richard Z. Hricak.

Got (Way Too Much) Milk?

Q:

While growing up, I was told that milk was the essential drink for staying healthy. Today, the advertisements from milk producers boast of vitamins, minerals, and, of course, calcium, calcium, calcium. In nature, milk is given to infants as a special diet to help them grow quickly. But is it healthy for adults?

A:

Much of the information that you've received about milk as "the essential drink" does come from the dairy industry, which has a vested interest in seeing that as many people as possible become lifetime consumers of milk and milk products.

In nature, animals drink milk only in infancy. And in many parts of the world, people react with disgust to the idea of drinking milk as adults. Milk is indeed a source of protein and calcium that some people do well on. But many adults have problems with one or more of its components.

Except among people of northern European origin, 75 percent of adults can't digest lactose, the sugar in milk. As they grow out of childhood, they stop making the enzyme that breaks down lactose. When lactose-intolerant people drink milk, they experience immediate digestive upsets: gas, cramps, and diarrhea.

Butterfat, the fat in milk, is the most saturated fat in the American diet. Cheese is often 70 percent—or more—fat by calories. Milk fat is a principal contributor to high cholesterol and atherosclerosis.

35

The protein in milk, casein, irritates the immune system in many people. This is the component of milk that stimulates mucus production as well. Casein is responsible for milk's association with conditions like recurrent ear infections in early life, eczema, chronic bronchitis, asthma, and sinusitis.

Most commercial milk also contains residues from drugs, hormones, and chemicals used to keep modern dairy cows producing abundantly.

I think most people should limit their intake of whole milk and the products made from it. Lactose-intolerant adults can eat cultured milk products (such as yogurt) now and then. To enjoy milk products occasionally without exposing yourself to so much fat, you can eat nonfat yogurt and mozzarella or other lowfat cheeses.

The dairy industry has done a great job convincing us that children are deprived without milk. I've kept my own five-year-old daughter off milk until recently. She has been remarkably healthy and has never had an ear infection.

I give her goat's milk, Rice Dream (which comes in different flavors), or a new product called DariFree. It's made from potatoes, and I think it's the best-tasting of the milk substitutes. The company has a toll-free information number: 800 275-1437. You should be aware that rice and potato drinks aren't protein-based. If you give any of these milk substitutes to your children, you'll also have to provide them with a different source of protein. (Soy milk does contain protein and is a good substitute for many people, but children are sometimes allergic to it.)

As for calcium, which helps regulate the nerves and muscles and is necessary for building strong bones, there are other ways to get it. Cooked greens (especially collards), molasses, sesame seeds, broccoli, and tofu are good sources.

How Bad
Is MSG?

Q:
How can MSG affect me?

A:
People react variably to monosodium glutamate, or MSG. Some people seem to be very sensitive to it, responding with nasal congestion, itching, flushing, headache, chest pain, and nausea. In its full-blown form, this reaction has been called "MSG symptom complex" by the medical establishment and "Chinese restaurant syndrome" by others.

MSG is found in many processed foods and ethnic cuisines. Chinese restaurants often add large amounts of it to stir-fried dishes. It's also used as a flavor enhancer in Japanese cooking, and it is common in packaged soups and sauces. The exact flavor MSG confers is difficult to describe; many just say it increases the "taste intensity" of food. One thing is certain: it makes people thirsty, encouraging them to eat and drink more. Americans consume about 28,000 tons of MSG per year, according to one estimate, reported in the *Journal of Environmental Health* (June 1995).

Chemically, MSG is one type of glutamate, a family of substances derived from glutamic acid, which in turn is one of the building blocks of proteins. "Free glutamate" like MSG is released by the breakdown of protein molecules. Some foods, including fresh tomatoes, tomato paste, and Parmesan cheese, naturally contain free glutamates. Monosodium glutamate was discovered in 1908 by Japanese researcher Kikunae Ikeda, who was looking for the flavor Japanese cooks prize in sea tangles, a type of sea vegetable. Scientists later learned to synthesize MSG as a pure crystalline substance.

Some doctors still dispute the existence of MSG symptom complex, while others believe it's an inherited allergic reaction. People who crusade against MSG cite a series of animal studies, using large amounts of MSG administered orally and by injection to rats and mice, that found the flavoring agent caused lesions in the hypothalamus, a vital brain center. But these studies represent extreme circumstances—the lesions didn't appear when MSG was added in normal amounts to the animals' diets—so they don't really provide any information about human consumption of MSG.

In 1995, a panel of experts convened by the Food and Drug Administration concluded that MSG doesn't cause any long-term medical problems. It did confirm that some people have strong short-term reactions within a half hour of eating three grams or more in a meal—about six times the amount you're likely to get in a single serving. The experts also found that people with severe asthma may suffer bronchospasms six to twelve hours after ingesting MSG, and that some individuals may react strongly even to very small amounts.

I have seen enough cases to convince me that MSG sensitivity is real. And when I go to Chinese restaurants (or others that might use MSG), I always ask to have the food prepared without it. Check the labels of the processed foods you eat for MSG; the manufacturer is required to list it on the label. Free glutamate is also present in various flavorings: hydrolyzed vegetable protein, calcium caseinate, sodium caseinate, soy sauce, and autolyzed yeast. Check the label for these as well. I don't know of any antidote to MSG, but one study has suggested that people who react to it are deficient in vitamin B-6; when they were given extra B-6 as a regular part of the diet, their symptoms didn't recur.

Just Say No to Laughing Gas?

Q:

Nitrous oxide—bad for the brain, or just clean fun?

A:

Nitrous oxide is also known as laughing gas. It got the name from traveling medicine shows and carnivals where the public would pay to inhale a minute's worth of the gas. People would laugh and act silly until the effect of the drug came to an abrupt end, when they would stand about in confusion. Yes, the good ol' days.

Nowadays, nitrous oxide is commonly used as a light general anesthetic for dental work and as a prelude to deeper anesthesia in surgery. It's also popular as a recreational drug to induce changes in consciousness or philosophical revelations, or just get hilariously intoxicated. The effects come on quickly and disappear just as fast.

Unfortunately, it isn't just clean fun. Nitrous oxide itself isn't bad for the brain, but unless you're careful in using it, you can deprive your brain of oxygen.

Some people breathe nitrous oxide straight out of tanks, a risky practice because you can asphyxiate yourself that way. Also, gas coming out of a pressurized tank is very cold and can cause frostbite of your nose, lips, or, most dangerously, larynx. Because of the anesthetic effects of the gas, you might not feel the damage until too late. The best way to avoid such dangers is to breathe nitrous oxide only from balloons—and only for a few minutes at a time.

Any way you breathe it, nitrous oxide can cause other serious injuries. People rapidly lose motor control under its influence and can fall over. So make sure you're sitting or lying down if you use it. It can also cause nausea and vomiting, particularly if you do it on a full stomach.

Regular use of nitrous oxide can impair fertility and interfere with the ability of the body to use vitamin B-12. A 1992 study published in the *New England Journal of Medicine* found that women exposed to high levels of nitrous oxide in their jobs (they were dental assistants) had a greater risk of infertility. Scientists speculate that the gas may interfere with the secretion of reproductive hormones. Interference with B-12 metabolism can result in damage to the bone marrow and nervous system. Loss of sensation in the feet and loss of balance may occur. I saw one patient, a man in his forties, who had developed severe pernicious anemia (vitamin B-12 deficiency) from breathing nitrous oxide on a regular basis and had those symptoms. It took a long time to clear up, even with regular vitamin B-12 shots.

What's Olestra All About?

Q:

I need info on olestra. What are the side effects? Does it take away nutrients from your system? I have heard that it flushes through the system and depletes vitamins. True?

A:

Olestra is a relatively new product that tastes and feels like fat but doesn't add fat or calories to the body because it's indigestible. The Center for Science in the Public Interest, a consumer group, asked the FDA to withdraw its approval of olestra because a study found that 20 percent of people who ate potato chips made with it had intestinal problems; for 3 percent of them, the problems were severe.

Olestra, manufactured by Procter & Gamble as Olean, is made with two natural products—sugar and vegetable oil. P & G replaces the glycerol in a normal fat with sucrose, then adds six, seven, or eight fatty acids instead of the three found in regular fat. What does this mean? Well, the resulting compound is too big to get into the bloodstream through the small intestine, so it really does flush through the system, as you say.

A one-ounce serving of regular potato chips contains about 150 calories and 10 grams (90 calories) of fat. Cooked in olestra, the same chips will contain about 70 calories and no fat.

The FDA approved olestra last year for use in potato chips, cheese puffs, crackers, and other salty snacks. P & G spent more than $200 million testing olestra to get it through regulatory scrutiny, but it is still under investigation for its long-term effects.

The studies found that olestra prevents absorption of vitamins A, D, E, and K, which hook onto the fat substitute and ride along as it passes through the intestine. The FDA required P & G to compensate by adding those vitamins to products containing olestra.

The fake fat also drags beta-carotene and other carotenoids along with it through the intestine and out of the body. Carotenoids may help prevent many kinds of cancer and other diseases, and some nutritionists have said they are concerned about the long-term impact of carotenoid loss due to olestra. Such questions are especially important since olestra could represent a significant change in the American diet, considering the quantities of fatty snacks people eat.

Other recorded side effects from olestra include bowel-function disruptions such as cramping, gas, diarrhea, and a problem euphemistically called "anal leakage."

The most pertinent question about olestra, though, is whether its benefits outweigh its potential hazards. Sugar substitutes haven't helped anyone lose weight. Whether fat substitutes will is not clear. I would say if you're going to consume olestra, do it moderately and cautiously until we have more information about it.

Poison on Your
Peaches?

Q:
I eat lots of fruits and veggies, but I'm worried about pesticides and other contaminants. What do you think?

A:
You are right to be worried. Not so long ago, hundreds of people in eight states and Toronto got sick after eating berries (originally reported to be strawberries, but now known to have been raspberries) contaminated with *Cyclospora*, a parasite that causes diarrhea, vomiting, weight loss, fatigue, and muscle aches. Investigators have speculated that harvesting crews passed along the parasite because they had no toilet facilities in the field, nor any place to wash their hands.

As to pesticides, although organic produce is becoming much more widely available and cheaper to buy, it's still a hassle to get it in most parts of the country. So, if it's not organic, it's important to know what you're eating. Always peel and wash fruits and vegetables, even though you can't rely on these practices to remove all pesticides. First, you won't affect any "systemic chemicals" that are taken up in a plant's roots and spread through its tissues. Second, other chemicals adhere so tightly to the plant or penetrate so deeply that they can't be washed away. Canned or frozen foods aren't an alternative, because it's the same sprayed fruit that goes into the packaging.

So it's important for you to know which crops are likely to carry the heaviest pesticide residues. Fruits to watch out for include apples, peaches, Chilean grapes, Mexican cantaloupes, strawberries, apricots, and cherries. Vegetables, grains, and legumes that are commonly contaminated include spinach, cucumbers, bell peppers, peanuts, green beans, potatoes, and wheat. The wax on the outside of apples, cucumbers, and green peppers usually contains fungicides. You have to peel these foods to remove the toxins.

In general, beware of imported fruit, which usually isn't checked very well to see if growers have met U.S. pesticide standards, which are much stricter than those in many other countries.

Your best bets are not to eat these crops at all, to grow your own, or to eat organic. You can grow a surprising amount of food in a very small space, and enjoy the emotional and physical benefits of gardening besides. Also, watch for pesticide-free displays in your supermarket, and get to know the laws in your state that govern when produce can be labeled organic. You can join consumer action groups to demand safe foods and clear labeling. Finally, find out about subscription or community agriculture, in which groups of consumers contract with growers to provide regular deliveries of organically produced fruits and vegetables.

I encourage people to support the organic agriculture movement, which is finally gaining a lot of ground in this country.

Let's Get a
Physical?

Q:
What would you recommend be included in an annual physical examination for a healthy forty-two-year-old? I've been trying to find information on this, but have been having trouble doing so.

A:
You don't say whether you're a man or a woman, so I'll answer for everyone. I'm not a believer in general physicals every year, but if you've never had a physical exam or haven't had one in a long while, get one. Even people in their twenties and thirties should get a complete check-up at some point as a baseline. General physicals become important as you enter your forties and fifties; then it makes sense to think about doing exams on a more regular basis.

The procedure should include a history—your description of your health history and any present problems—a physical examination by a doctor, and standard lab tests. It's important that you talk to your doctor about any concerns you have about your health. You might want to bring a list of questions. (In addition to physical symptoms, you should talk to your doctor about any emotional or psychological difficulties.) Remember, most doctors work under factory-like conditions these days, and you've got to make sure you get the attention you need. Be an assertive patient!

There are standard assessments that should be included in every physical exam and other tests that may be appropriate, depending on your medical history. Usually the doctor will start by recording your height, weight, pulse, and blood pressure, then check your heart, lungs, lymph nodes, and abdomen.

For anyone in his or her forties, the visit should include a rectal examination, plus a stool sample to test for blood. For women, the exam should include a breast and vaginal examination and a Pap smear (to check for cancer of the cervix). Women should have an annual breast exam, pelvic exam, and Pap smear.

There is also a standard battery of blood tests that should be done, including a complete blood count and an SMAC 20. I would also include a complete lipid panel to measure cholesterol and blood fats. Your urine should be sampled for testing, too.

Men over fifty should have a serum PSA (prostate specific antigen) test, which screens for prostate cancer, and an electrocardiogram (EKG). Women should have a mammogram at age forty.

Eyeing Plastic Surgery?

Q:

I am thinking about having cosmetic surgery on my eyelids. I am only in my late twenties, but I have to do it because my eyelids really drag down. I don't know what I will look like afterward; all I can imagine is how horrific I am going to look with the stitches in. I have asked the plastic surgeon for some pictures, but he says he doesn't have any. What can I do about this anxiety, and the shock I will get when I see my eyes like that?

A:

First, please don't agree to have cosmetic surgery without really thinking it through carefully—not just about what it may look like along the way and afterward, but also about what you expect from it and why you want it. Be sure you really want this procedure. Ask your surgeon to explain in detail all the things that can go wrong. Find out what results the surgery can and can't give you. If your surgeon can't or won't tell you, look for a different one. I've written before about the importance of being an assertive patient; it is especially important when you are considering elective surgery. The cost for upper and lower lids can be as much as $7,000, and that won't be covered by your insurance provider.

As for your immediate concerns, you're right: you have to be prepared for the week or two after surgery when you'll look worse than you did before it. It will take five to eight weeks until you're completely healed. A good resource for anyone considering plastic surgery is Diana Barry's *Nips & Tucks: Everything You Must Know Before Having Cosmetic Surgery*.

Barry covers everything from eyelid surgery to collagen injections and postmastectomy breast reconstruction.

Other, more invasive procedures—like face-lifts—can take even more time to heal fully (and can leave you with permanent side effects). I've seen some very good results from cosmetic surgery. But I've also seen a number of cases where faces ended up looking very unnatural, with the skin appearing stretched, for example.

I don't know if you smoke. People who smoke tobacco are at higher risk for complications from cosmetic surgery, because they have decreased blood circulation in the skin. If you can't quit altogether, your surgeon will suggest stopping ten days before surgery, and for a week post-op. That's the minimum.

I also have to say that all this sounds premature. You said you're in your twenties, which is very young to be considering cosmetic surgery. Ask yourself a few basic questions before you do anything else. Why aren't you happy with yourself as you are? Is your unhappiness with your eyelids reflective of a larger dissatisfaction with yourself? Does your decision to change your eyelids rest on what other people have been telling you about your appearance? Maybe there are ways other than surgery for you to become happier. How about talking over the possibilities with a counselor before going further?

Find the
Right Shrink?

Q:

The psychiatrist I was seeing retired after just three visits, and I began to see another doctor a month ago. My question now is, is it better to see a psychiatrist or a psychoanalyst? One of my main problems is dependency. I can't seem to make decisions without the approval or support of someone. I was told that besides giving you Xanax for anxiety, a psychiatrist tends to listen more and let you figure out your own problems, and an analyst becomes more involved in discussion with the patient. Which is better for me?

A:

The bottom line for mental-health care is really a matter of what you can afford, how much time you want to devote to the problem, and, most important, the chemistry between you and the counselor you choose.

Managed care has changed the way mental-health services are provided. Because of time constraints and limits on the number of visits allowed, more mental-health providers now lean toward drug therapy instead of problem-solving sessions. Most health plans cover only a few visits a year, and will pay no more than $50,000 in mental-health care over a lifetime. On first glance that may seem like a lot, but the dollar amount also encompasses hospitalization for serious mental illnesses, which is expensive.

Psychiatrists are M.D.s, and they can prescribe medication. Their medical training has concentrated on the treatment and prevention of mental, emotional, and behavioral disorders. Psychoanalysts are a special subclass of psychiatrists with additional training who subscribe to Sigmund Freud's theories and try to help you become aware of unconscious drives that affect behavior. Generally, the psychoanalyst sits out of sight while the patient reclines on a couch, recounting dreams, describing childhood incidents, and free-associating. Many try to inject themselves as little as possible into the unfolding of the patient's unconscious. Psychoanalysis is very time- and cost-intensive, and is sharply declining in popularity.

Psychologists and licensed clinical social workers engage in interactive counseling, helping the patient unravel the interaction between buried drives, past history, and physical and social environment; often, they turn to dreams and childhood memories as tools. More and more, the lines are becoming blurred between the different specialists. Managed care is encouraging streamlined approaches to all these interventions.

There are many subspecialties within each of the fields. Your best bet is to try out several people and see with whom you feel most comfortable. Ask them about the theories they use, the political ideologies they may apply, what they charge, what health plans they accept, and anything else that seems important to you. Ask what sessions with them will be like, and how long they think treatment may take.

It may be that you should be on medication, though I wouldn't want you to jump to that conclusion because you feel anxiety. There are other effective methods to relieve anxious feelings, and only someone who sees you in person and talks with you at length can help you decide what's best. Even then, it may require some experimentation.

Xanax, or alprazolam, is an addictive drug that can interfere with mental function, so you may want to consider alternative treatments before you start taking it. A natural remedy for anxiety is tincture of passionflower (*Passiflora incarnata*), which is mildly relaxing. The dose is one dropperful in a little water up to four times a day, as needed. Tincture of valerian (*Valeriana officianalis*) is more powerful—

use 10 to 15 drops in water up to four times a day as needed. I also recommend trying my relaxing breathing exercise (see page 62).

Radiation Dangers from Household Appliances?

Q:
I see a lot of news about radiation emitted by everything from cellular phones to radios to electric blankets. What are your opinions regarding the risks from these devices?

A:
Much has been written about the dangers of electric clock radios, electric blankets, heating pads, and hair dryers. All of these appliances generate electromagnetic fields that can disrupt delicate body control systems, possibly increasing the risk of cancer and weakening immunity. I wouldn't keep an electric clock radio near my head, and I wouldn't use any of these appliances on a regular basis. The best source of information about household radiation is *Cross Currents* by Robert O. Becker, M.D.

As for cellular phones, most of the scientists and all the manufacturers say there's nothing of concern here, despite the media furor. I have seen ads for shields that you can slip over the phone to block any radiation. If you're worried, do that.

Microwave ovens are generally safe; they rarely leak radiation, unless damaged. But they can alter the chemistry of protein foods cooked in them for long periods of time as well as drive foreign molecules into food wrapped in plastic wrap or cooked in plastic containers.

(Some cooking tips: Use microwaves for defrosting and quick heating, rather than long cooking of main dishes. Always use glass or ceramic containers to cook in. Never use plastic wrap during cooking.)

Everyone I've spoken to says that the new generation of computer monitors present little risk or hazard. Most of the radiation comes out of the back—a fact you should be aware of. I used to use a computer monitor shield, but with a more recent model I don't. Because radiation falls off exponentially with distance, it never hurts to put a little more distance between you and the source.

Is Radon
Really Dangerous?

Q:

How dangerous is radon? We have lived for over fifteen years in a house that has from 17 to 28 picocuries per liter of radon in the basement, where our family room, computer room, and playroom are located. My husband doesn't want to spend the money to get rid of the radon.

A:

Radon is a natural radioactive element produced by the decay of radium in the Earth's crust. It's an odorless, colorless gas that seeps out of the earth, more commonly in some places on the planet than others. It sometimes enters the basements of houses through cracks and pipes and becomes trapped there, concentrated in the air we breathe.

Radon is strongly carcinogenic, and is believed to be the second leading cause of lung cancer—after cigarette smoking. It may account for as many as 30,000 deaths a year in the United States. Radon is dangerous, but I don't think anyone can say exactly how dangerous. You can have the air in your house tested for radon, but if there's a high level, it's not clear what you should do.

Check with your regional office of the Environmental Protection Agency. Those folks can tell you how serious your problem may be and which ventilation systems work best. You also can get information on test kits and ways to reduce gas levels through the National Safety Council's National Radon Hotline at 800 767-7236.

You can install an exhaust system, which may remove the

radon from the air coming into the basement. You can also cover and seal drains, pipes, and cracks in the foundation, where the radon could be leaking in. If the level stays at 4 pico-curies per liter (pCi/L) or higher and you are concerned, you may want to move to another house. Obviously, that's easier said than done.

The bottom line: Radon is dangerous, and if there's a significant level of it in your house, I think you and your husband should spend the money to do something about it.

Red Wine for
a Healthy Heart?

Q:
What are the pros and cons of drinking red wine?

A:
The wine industry has benefited tremendously from reports that moderate drinking of red wine can lower the risk of coronary heart disease. After *60 Minutes* reported on the "French Paradox" in 1991, sales of cabernet and merlot soared.

The French Paradox was first discovered when epidemiologists tried to explain the lower-than-expected death rates from heart disease in France in spite of a high-fat, high-cholesterol diet. Various studies followed that showed an association between drinking red wine and a heart attack risk that was 25 to 40 percent lower. *60 Minutes* followed up with a report from the Copenhagen City Heart Study of 13,000 people over ten years: the researchers had concluded that teetotalers had twice as much risk of dying from heart disease as people who drank wine every day.

The exact mechanism isn't known, but the most popular explanation credits the red pigments in grape skins. These pigments belong to a family of compounds called proanthocyanidins, which are powerful antioxidants that may protect arteries from circulating cholesterol. If this is the primary action, you could get the same benefits from drinking red grape juice or eating enough red and purple fruit. In fact, more recent research makes red grape juice look even more protective than red wine.

The tannins in red wine as well as the alcohol can keep

platelets in the blood from clumping together and triggering a heart attack. Plus, studies have found that any alcohol can raise levels of HDL—the good form of cholesterol that prevents arterial damage.

But let's not forget that alcohol is toxic to the liver and nervous system. The French have a higher risk of liver disease. Most wines also contain a variety of additives, such as sulfites, which may be unhealthy. If you're going to be a regular wine drinker, I'd recommend moderation. I'd also look for organic products. Both domestic and imported organic wines of good quality are becoming more available.

I don't drink red wine because it gives me a stuffy nose and a morning-after sour stomach—probably reactions to additives or constituents other than alcohol. Red wine is a common allergen that can trigger migraine headaches as well as nasal and gastric disturbances.

Is Rolfing Better than Massage?

Q:
I'd like to know your opinions on Rolfing and if you think it is a more beneficial form of massage than others. Thanks.

A:
Rolfing is not simply massage. It's a form of body work intended to restructure the connective tissue, or fascia. Basic Rolfing consists of ten intensive sessions in which the practitioner applies firm—even painful—pressure with the fingers and elbows to specific parts of the body. For people who are open to Rolfing, it can be a great way to get more in touch with your body and change long-standing problems of bad posture and chronic pain (like back pain). Rolfing can also release repressed emotions as well as diminish habitual muscle tension. If you want to make some kind of change in your life and work on your body, you might consider Rolfing. For a referral in your area, contact the Rolf Institute (see Other Resources, page 80).

Sauna Making
You Sweat?

Q:

I've heard totally varied opinions on the benefits/hazards of saunas and steam baths. What's your opinion?

A:

To me, the benefits far outweigh the hazards. If you're in reasonable health, the benefits of a sauna or steam bath are great. If you have high blood pressure or heart disease, saunas may be good for you, but you'll want to be cautious; check with your physician first, and go slow. And with either of these conditions, it's not a good idea to jump right into cold water afterward, as Finns do.

When you take a sauna, the heat pumps up blood circulation near the skin and stimulates sweating. The Finns say a proper sauna elicits about a quart of sweat per hour. I generally encourage sweating, because it helps the body rid itself of unwanted materials. In medieval times, healers relied on sweat baths to cure illnesses, and priests used them to chase away evil spirits.

American physicians usually warn pregnant women not to take steam baths or saunas. A study published in 1992 in the *Journal of the American Medical Association* found some association between neural tube defects and heat exposure from saunas, hot tubs, and fever during the first three months of pregnancy. (Neural tube defects include anencephaly and spina bifida, both disastrous fetal abnormalities.) The biggest problem was posed by hot tubs, which pregnant women should definitely approach with caution.

Interestingly, though, in Finland it's not uncommon for doctors to give the OK on saunas from conception all the way up to the day of delivery—and there, neural tube defects are very low. In fact, in Finland saunas were once a traditional place for childbirth. It's worth noting that Finnish women tend to stay in the sauna for six to twelve minutes, and they shorten that time during pregnancy. Also, even though they feel very hot, saunas raise the body's core temperature insignificantly compared to hot tubs.

Finnish saunas are different from most U.S. versions—unless these are run by Scandinavians. In Finland, saunas are usually heated by a wood stove. First there's a dry phase that can get hotter than 200° F. Then the participants splash water on the stove and spend some time in the steam. Many U.S. saunas employ an electric stove, which you can't put water on. So you're just exposed to dry heat, which I, for one, find irritating to my respiratory passages. Some saunas in health clubs are set to a lukewarm temperature. Turn up the heat.

Even if you're in a very hot steam bath or sauna, it's mostly the temperature of the surface of your body that goes up. As it does so, blood vessels dilate, and circulation increases in the skin. As resistance to blood flow through your veins and capillaries drops, your blood pressure goes down. Then your heartbeat increases to keep blood pressure normal.

Finns always follow a sauna with a plunge into cold water. This is incredibly refreshing and enjoyable. Then you relax.

The main risk of a sauna is staying in too long and fainting from overheating. People who are most susceptible are those with heart disease and those who have been using drugs or alcohol. It isn't a good idea to combine alcohol and other drugs with saunas or hot tubs. Also, be sure you drink plenty of water, to replace the water you're losing. Children should not use saunas or hot tubs without supervision.

By the way, the correct pronunciation is *sow-na*, not *saw-na*.

Commit to
Quit Smoking?

Q:
I know I should quit. I just can't seem to. I desperately need help.

A:
Many smokers stare at themselves in the mirror, asking, "How do I quit?" It's hard. Tobacco, in the form of cigarettes, is the most addictive drug in the world—right up there with crack cocaine. There are two reasons for this: Nicotine is one of the strongest stimulants known, and smoking is one of the most efficient drug-delivery systems. Smoking actually puts drugs into the brain more directly than intravenous injection.

In the early part of this century, cigarette smoking was accepted, and was even considered healthy and glamorous. It was thought to promote mental acuity, efficiency, and relaxation. It is true that one of the "benefits" of smoking is a brief relief of internal tension; unfortunately, within twenty minutes the tension is back stronger than before, and the brain demands another fix.

Low-tar, low-nicotine cigarettes offer no great advantages. People tend to smoke more of them, or inhale more deeply to get the same amount of nicotine. Pipes and cigars, if the smoke is not inhaled, do not cause lung cancer and emphysema, but they do increase the risk of oral cancer (as do snuff and chewing tobacco).

I feel so strongly about the health risks of smoking that I will not accept patients who are users unless they are willing to try to quit. Many programs can help you: acupuncture, hypnotherapy, and support groups. There are also a slew of new devices on the market—nicotine patches and gum, for instance—that work for some. None of these methods works reliably for everyone. Most successful quitters do it on their own after one or more unsuccessful attempts. Going "cold turkey" also seems to work better than gradually cutting down.

Don't get discouraged. If you can't quit today, you may be able to tomorrow. Motivation is the key, and it can come only from you. Remember: You get credit for every attempt you make. In fact, the best predictor for success is making attempts to quit.

If you smoke, do this breathing exercise. It will help motivate you to quit and help you with your cravings for cigarettes when you do. Here's how:

1. Sit with your back straight. Place the tip of your tongue against the ridge of tissue behind your upper front teeth, and keep it there throughout the exercise.
2. Exhale completely through your mouth, making a *whoosh* sound.
3. Close your mouth and inhale quietly through your nose to a silent count of four.
4. Hold your breath for a count of seven.
5. Exhale completely through your mouth, again making a *whoosh* sound, to a count of eight.
6. This is one breath. Now inhale again and repeat the cycle three more times.

Do this throughout the day, whenever you crave a smoke.

If you smoke, you should take antioxidant vitamins and minerals, which to some extent can reverse the changes in respiratory tissue caused by tobacco, and so help protect against lung cancer. Also, increase your intake of dietary sources of carotenes (carrots, sweet potatoes, yellow and orange squash and fruits, and leafy green vegetables).

Good luck, and please set a date for your next attempt to quit.

Additive-Free Sports Drinks?

Q:

Do you know of any energy drinks that are a bit lighter on the chemicals and better for you than Gatorade and the like? I am a runner and I enjoy these drinks but wonder if there isn't something out there that is better for me.

A:

I don't usually recommend commercial energy drinks, because they contain artificial dyes and other unhealthy additives.

When you exercise, you lose a lot of fluids and some minerals from exertion. Fluid loss can be major, especially if you're running in a hot climate or for longer than an hour. And dehydration can drastically impair performance and mental sharpness.

Energy drinks help most because they contain water, simple sugars, and electrolytes such as sodium and potassium. There's also evidence that drinking one of these before exercising may boost your ability to work out harder and longer, as long as you're doing something that doesn't require a lot of stops and starts. These drinks bring your blood sugar up to its normal operating range as you start to work out; while you're exercising, hormonal changes keep it steady. (If you stop or slow down significantly, your blood sugar may spike, and then fall when you start your workout again.) A caution: Don't use these drinks more than a few minutes before exercising, or you may feel a sharp drop in blood sugar once you start.

Whatever you do, drink lots of water. Drink more than you think you need. Studies have shown that recreational runners tend to drink less than they need—before, during, and after exercise. If you've lost a lot of salt or potassium from exercise, you can replace those substances by eating some fruits or vegetables. I don't know that there's a need for any kind of sports drink after exercise. But if you enjoy such drinks, look for natural versions that don't have additives and artificial colors. Health food stores carry them. Or you can make your own.

Natural Sports Drink

Over medium heat, dissolve $\frac{1}{4}$ cup sugar in 2 cups of water. Add $\frac{1}{4}$ tsp salt. Remove from stove, cool, and add $\frac{1}{4}$ cup of orange juice. Mix with water to fill a quart bottle—and go!

Are Steroids Okay?

Q:

What's your opinion of steroids and protein drinks to enhance athletic performance?

A:

I'm opposed to the use of both kinds of products.

Anabolic steroids are sex hormones, usually synthetic, that increase protein metabolism, bone density, and muscle bulk. For some time, male athletes and bodybuilders have been taking anabolic steroids to build muscles and enhance performance. In fact, this practice is astonishingly common. Five years ago, the Drug Enforcement Administration made anabolic steroids controlled substances, ending legal prescription of them, but other sources have appeared. The promise of rapid development of big muscles and a powerful body image is very seductive, especially to teens and young men.

A study published July 4, 1996, in *The New England Journal of Medicine* reported that injections of testosterone (a natural anabolic steroid) added extra muscle and strength in a group of 40 male bodybuilders. *The New York Times* headline put it succinctly: TESTOSTERONE = BIG MUSCLES. That's not news, really. What's important to ask is: What's the downside?

There's plenty to talk about. It is widely accepted that steroids can have very significant adverse effects, including loss of sexual potency and drive and erratic mood swings. They also increase your risk of heart disease and high blood pressure and can cause acne, baldness, and abnormal liver function. Women may experience masculinizing changes, such

65

as a deepened voice and increased facial hair. In fact, women were excluded from the recent study, because the potential side effects for them were considered unacceptable.

Proponents of steroids say these effects are rare. They will be encouraged by the *New England Journal of Medicine* study, which also found no evidence that steroids made the weight lifters more aggressive. I think it's important to note that the study was of short duration (ten weeks) and the dose of testosterone given was much lower than what most bodybuilders take.

In my view, steroids unbalance the body's hormonal system and ultimately lead to weakening of the body. High doses may be addictive.

As for protein supplements, I can see no reason to use them. I've seen competitive bodybuilders who developed liver dysfunction as a result of force-feeding on protein. Excess consumption of protein—in any form—puts an added workload on the digestive system, liver, and kidneys. Protein is not a very efficient fuel for the body. It takes more energy to digest and metabolize, and it breaks down into toxic residues that the liver and kidneys must handle. The breakdown products of protein metabolism can also irritate the immune system.

Blocking Sunburn Damage?

Q:
After shaving my head I spent a weekend in the Rocky Mountain sun. Despite putting on an SPF-30 sunscreen, I woke up Monday morning with a blistering, crusty, pus-spewing top. Now it's better and the skin is just peeling, but do I have anything to be concerned about?

A:
Ouch.

The incidence of skin cancer is rising at an alarming rate, with ultraviolet (UV) radiation from the sun the major cause. One reason may be the weakening of the Earth's protective ozone layer as a result of atmospheric pollution, so that more solar radiation is now reaching us. Even though UV waves are longer and have less energy than ionizing radiation like X rays, they are still powerful enough to penetrate living cells in the skin and cause DNA damage. UV radiation doesn't just hurt the skin; it can also cause loss of vision as you grow older by damaging the retina (macular degeneration) and the lens (cataract).

I always recommend protecting yourself in as many ways as possible. Stay out of the sun when it's at a high angle in the sky. Choose clothing that covers your skin—brimmed hats, lightweight, long-sleeve shirts. Use a powerful sunscreen (SPF-15, at least) that blocks both UVA and UVB, and wear UV-protective sunglasses. And, finally, take antioxidants to help block the chemical reactions that can lead to cancer. Living in the Arizona desert, I try to follow this advice year-round.

Cancer risks increase with cumulative exposure, so you should definitely avoid getting another burn on your head. The more bad burns you get, especially in your teenage years and in your twenties, the higher your risk of skin cancer as you age. If you stop getting burned, you will lessen the danger.

Most dermatologists say it's a good idea to get in the habit of putting a high-SPF sunscreen on every morning. I agree. But as you've found, sunscreen can give you a false sense of protection. Just because you're wearing sunscreen, don't assume you can spend unlimited time in the sun. It's still good to be careful. You got in trouble because you were at a high altitude, where thinner atmosphere lets more UV radiation in. You needed even more protection than your sunscreen gave you.

An old-fashioned sunscreen that is still effective is zinc oxide. This is an opaque cream that provides a mechanical barrier to sunlight. (It's now available in neon colors as well as in the original white.) It works extremely well if you don't mind walking around with your face completely white or electric blue.

If you do get burned, aloe is probably the most soothing treatment. You can buy bottles of the pure gel in health food stores or grow the plants around your house.

Burning for
a Quick Tan?

Q:

How bad is it to self-tan? Is it any better for you than the sun?

A:

People can't seem to get away from the idea that a tan is healthy and beautiful. That's why there are self-tanning lotions and tanning salons.

The lotions are harmless, but the results never quite look natural to me. Fortunately, there are now improved formulas that at least don't leave you streaked with orange. The new products contain dehydroxyacetone, which interacts with proteins in the surface cells of your skin. Some people complain about a slight chemical or metallic scent, but that goes away in a few hours.

To avoid blotches, you need to be careful when applying the lotion. First, get rid of dry, flaky skin with a sponge or washcloth. Remove your rings and other jewelry, and apply the tanner lightly just as you would a body lotion. Put only a little on your knees and elbows—the dry skin will absorb more color than the rest of your body. Try not to get the lotion under your nails, since it will discolor them, and wash your hands immediately so your palms don't look unnaturally tan. Then, remember that even though your skin is more brown, it's not protected by the melanin produced by a natural suntan. So be sure to use lots of sunscreen before going out in the sun. Apply the sunscreen only after the tanning lotion is completely dry.

As for tanning salons, my advice is to stay away. The rays in a tanning parlor can actually be stronger than ordinary sunshine. A study in Sweden a couple of years ago found that people under age thirty who used tanning salons more than ten times a year had a seven times higher risk of melanoma than other people. Most skin cancer is related to UV radiation, and melanoma is the deadliest kind. There's no such thing as "tanning" rays, as distinct from "burning" rays. The UV-A light of tanning salons is at least as harmful as the UV-B rays you get during peak sunlight hours.

Sometimes people go to tanning salons before they go on a winter vacation in order to avoid a sunburn. A better technique is to expose yourself gradually to the sun once you've arrived, and be sure to use a sunblock of at least SPF-15.

I'm not one of those doctors who would have you avoid sun at any cost, but a tan is definitely not a sign of health. The only good thing about a suntan is that it means you've been outdoors, where you may have been getting exercise, relaxing, and having fun. To get tan in a shop, without the associated healthful activities, is not quite what the doctor ordered.

Is My Toothbrush Alive?

Q:
I'm concerned about bacteria or whatever growing on my toothbrush. How often would you advise changing to a new toothbrush? Is it advisable to disinfect a toothbrush between uses, perhaps by soaking it in salt solution?

A:
First of all, never exchange toothbrushes with another person. That's an easy way to spread colds and other infections. In particular, it's possible to contract hepatitis B, C, or D if you share a toothbrush with someone who's already infected. Virus-infected blood and bodily fluids are the known modes of transmission. HIV can also be transmitted by sharing personal items like toothbrushes and razors (through infected blood, not saliva). Bottom line: It's always better to spend the extra buck or two and get a new toothbrush rather than share. Keep an extra in your medicine cabinet.

With your own toothbrush, bacteria won't be that much of a problem if you use a toothpaste with an antibacterial agent like tea tree oil (from the leaves of *Melaleuca alternifolia*) or chlorine dioxide in it. Just go ahead and air dry the brush in a place that's fairly sanitary—away from the toilet, for example, and not in the trajectory of splashes from the sink.

It's good to change toothbrushes fairly frequently—say, every two or three months. This will keep your brushing effective, in addition to keeping your toothbrush cleaner.

While we're on the subject, here are some brushing basics: Use a brush with soft bristles, so you don't damage your teeth or gums. Brush gently at least twice a day, holding your toothbrush at a 45-degree angle. Use small circular motions. Scrubbing your tongue will get rid of bacteria and freshen your breath. Remember: To avoid damaging your gums, don't brush too hard.

Electric toothbrushes sound great but I've never grown to like any of them. Some dentists love the ultrasonic ones that emit inaudible high-frequency sound waves to kill bacteria while you're brushing. Use these appliances if you want, but a plain old manual toothbrush does the job just fine.

Don't forget to floss!

Walking for Your Life?

Q:

Is it true that walking is almost equal to jogging as an aerobic exercise?

A:

I'm a great proponent of walking. Not only is it almost equal to jogging in terms of getting your heart pumping, but I think research eventually will show that it's superior in terms of overall health benefits. There are many reasons to prefer walking to just about any other form of exercise. First of all, everyone knows how to do it and it doesn't require any equipment. Second, you can do it anywhere. Third, the risk of injury is far less than for any other kind of aerobic exercise.

With running, the risk of injury is high. Runners who go for endorphin highs often run through warning pain—then wind up being unable to exercise at all. They may also become exercise addicts.

I sometimes take a morning walk after I meditate. Or in the afternoon, I might walk around the ranch where I live. If I'm in a city like New York or San Francisco, I try to do as much walking as possible. San Francisco is great because of the hills, and in New York the people-watching always keeps me entertained.

You may find walking meditative and relaxing. As you do it, you can take in the sights or listen to something on a Walkman. Walking exercises your brain as well as your body; its cross-patterned movement (right arm moves forward with the left leg) generates harmonizing electrical activity in your brain.

73

I find that good running shoes with cushioned soles are best for walking. But experiment—find out what works for you. If you walk up a long, gradual hill or walk at a good clip, you can get your heart and respiratory rates high enough to produce the aerobic conditioning you need. Maintain good posture and be sure to swing your arms as you go. I recommend forty-five minutes of walking a day. That's about three miles. Do it at least five times a week.

What's the Best Water Filter?

Q:

I know there are a lot of contaminants and toxins in water these days. What do you recommend for a water filter?

A:

Water quality varies from place to place, so you should have your water tested to see what impurities it contains. The results will help you decide whether you actually need a filter and what type to get. Note that it can cost more than $100 to test for a range of contaminants.

Chlorine and lead are the two most common problems. Chlorine is a powerful oxidizing agent that can cause birth defects, cancer, and heart disease. As for lead, even very small amounts can be harmful, especially to young children. Lead poisoning causes organ damage and stunts the nervous system, producing mental retardation.

In many cities, public health officials are also finding *Cryptosporidium* in water; this is a microbe that can cause great harm to people with compromised immune systems.

Check out the different kinds of filtration systems available, making sure to find out how often you need to change filters, how much the replacements cost, and how difficult they are to install. Systems vary in quality, efficiency, and price.

Six systems are available for purifying water at home. None of them is perfect. Each has distinct strengths and drawbacks. Always read the labeling to learn exactly what the product claims to remove.

Steam distillation is the surest method. Water is heated to

boiling, the steam collected and cooled until it condenses again without the impurities. This method works, but it's the most expensive one. Distillation will not remove a few volatile organic compounds, which boil over with the steam.

Carbon filtration is probably the most popular system. Units containing specially prepared, porous carbon attach under the sink or at the tap. Carbon filtration is good for removing chlorine, toxic organic molecules, and bad tastes from water, but it doesn't capture heavy metals or minerals. The system is fast, but it stops working as soon as the carbon becomes saturated with contaminants. Also, as the carbon collects organic matter, it becomes a breeding ground for bacteria. Bacteria will pour out into your first glass of water of the day, unless you take a minute to flush the filter first.

Ion-exchange rids water of dissolved minerals and toxic metals, but it is less efficient at removing organic molecules. It works through charged particles in the filter that exchange themselves for charged particles in the water. These filters normally employ sodium in the exchange, so unless there's another process to remove it later, you could end up with harmful levels of sodium in the purified water. Water purified by this method will corrode pipes, carrying metals out of them. I don't recommend it.

Purifiers that use ultraviolet light to kill microorganisms have no effect on chemical contaminants.

In the past, I used a system called reverse osmosis (RO). RO removes minerals and toxic metals like lead, along with organic contaminants (and *Cryptosporidium*). In an RO unit, water pressure forces water through an osmotic membrane (one with tiny holes that allow small water molecules, but not contaminant molecules, to pass through). Bacteria are blocked, and they don't grow on the filter. This may be the best way to go. However, you should know that the process is slow, and wastes a lot of water, which is why I finally stopped using it. I can't afford to waste water in the desert. RO water is also very corrosive to pipes, so place the system near the tap.

A newer system that looks good combines a solid carbon block filter with a copper-zinc alloy called KDF. This dual cartridge system removes most impurities and is affordable and simple. The KDF puts small amounts of copper and zinc into the water, which most experts consider healthful.

Resources

Books by Andrew Weil, M.D.

8 Weeks to Optimum Health: A Proven Program for Taking Full Advantage of Your Body's Natural Healing Power. New York: Alfred A. Knopf, 1997.

Spontaneous Healing: How to Discover and Enhance Your Body's Natural Ability to Maintain and Heal Itself. New York: Ballantine Books, 1996.

Natural Health, Natural Medicine: A Comprehensive Manual for Wellness and Self-Care. Rev. ed. Boston: Houghton Mifflin, 1995.

Health and Healing: Understanding Conventional and Alternative Medicine. Rev. ed. Boston: Houghton Mifflin, 1995.

From Chocolate to Morphine: Everything You Need to Know About Mind-Altering Drugs, with Winifred Rosen. Rev. ed. Boston: Houghton Mifflin, 1993.

The Natural Mind: An Investigation of Drugs and the Higher Consciousness. Rev. ed. Boston: Houghton Mifflin, 1986.

The Marriage of the Sun and the Moon: A Quest for Unity in Consciousness. Boston: Houghton Mifflin, 1980.

Other Recommended Books

Barry, Diana. *Nips & Tucks: Everything You Must Know Before Having Cosmetic Surgery.* Los Angeles: General Publishing Group, 1996.

Becker, Robert O. *Cross Currents: The Perils of Electropollution, the Promise of Electromedicine.* Los Angeles: Jeremy Tarcher, 1990; dist. by St. Martin's Press.

Washnis, George J., and Richard Z. Hricak. *Discovery of Magnetic Health: A Health Care Alternative.* Rockville, Maryland: Nova Publishing, 1993.

Other Resources

American Association of Naturopathic Physicians
601 Valley Street, Suite 105
Seattle, WA 98109
206 298-0125

Heintzman Farms
R.R. 2, Box 265
Onaka, SD 57466
605 447-5813

EPA Safe Drinking Water Hotline
800 426-4791

National Radon Hotline
800 767-7236

Rolf Institute
205 Canyon Boulevard
Boulder, CO 80302
303 449-5903 or 800 530-8875
Fax: 303 449-5978

Program in Integrative Medicine

At the University of Arizona Health Sciences Center, Tucson, Arizona. For more information, visit the Web site: http://www.ahsc.arizona.edu/integrative_medicine. Or write: Center for Integrative Medicine, P.O. Box 64089, Tucson, AZ 85718.

Newsletter

If you would like information on my lectures and informational products, including my monthly newsletter, *Self Healing*, please write to: Andrew Weil, M.D., P.O. Box 457, Vail, AZ 85641.

On the Web

"Ask Dr. Weil" answers health questions daily on Time Warner's Pathfinder Network (www.drweil.com).

Index

About Andrew Weil, M.D.

Dr. Andrew Weil is the leader in the new field of Integrative Medicine, which combines the best ideas and practices of conventional and alternative medicine. A graduate of Harvard Medical School, he is director of the Program in Integrative Medicine at the University of Arizona, the first program to train physicians in this way at an American medical school. He is also the founder of the Center for Integrative Medicine in Tucson, which is advancing the field worldwide. Dr. Weil is well known as an expert in natural medicine, mind-body interactions, and medical botany, as well as the author of the bestselling *Spontaneous Healing* and *8 Weeks to Optimum Health.* According to Dr. Weil, "Spontaneous healing is not a miracle or a lucky exception, but a fact of biology, the result of the natural healing system that each of us is born with."

About "Ask Dr. Weil"

The "Ask Dr. Weil" program (www.drweil.com) features Andrew Weil, M.D., and is one of the top-rated health sites on the World Wide Web and is featured on Time Warner's Pathfinder Network. The recipient of many awards, the "Ask Dr. Weil" program features a daily Q&A with answers to a wide range of health questions, a daily poll, and the Doc Weil Database, which lets readers search hundreds of topics, including material from Dr. Weil's bestselling book *Natural Health, Natural Medicine.* The site also features a Referral Directory (practitioners from acupuncture to Trager work) and DocTalk, a live weekly chat with Dr. Weil. If you have additional questions for Dr. Weil, ask them on his Web site.

About Steven Petrow (Series Editor)

Steven Petrow is the executive producer of the "Ask Dr. Weil" program. Mr. Petrow has held editorial positions with *Life* magazine, *Longevity* magazine, *Fitness*, and *The Wall Street Journal*. He's also been the editor-in-chief of *10 Percent* magazine and *AIDS Digest* and has published five books, including *The HIV Drug Book* and *When Someone You Know Has AIDS*.

Acknowledgments

Richard Pine, Judith Curr, Elisa Wares, and Scott Fagan